Coconut Paradise

Coconut Milk, Oil and Flour

Cookbook

A Delicious and Low-Calorie Alternative to Fatty Foods

Disclaimer

Table of Contents

Summary

Coconut is one of those tropical treats which not only serve the mere purpose of a fruit, but it also assists a great deal in fat free cooking. For years, people have been raving about the health benefits of coconut oil and milk, but recent studies have also proved that replacing cereal flour with coconut flour can considerably help in regard to people's weight in a healthy way. If you are looking for an inclusive guide to help you make the most of this amazing fruit, you have come to the right place.

This eBook informs readers about the health benefits of consuming coconut milk, coconut flour and coconut water on a regular basis. Moreover, readers can also find 23 amazing coconut oil and 17 coconut flour recipes and 16 coconut milk recipes. These recipes are not only easy to make but also delicious. Unlike other health guides, this eBook contains breakfast, snack, lunch and dinner recipes, thus offering readers a complete coconut platter.

The eBook also informs readers about the calorie content and preparation time of each dish. You can also find health benefits of coconut oil, flour and milk, and how daily intake of coconut in various forms can cure several diseases.

If you are tired of the taste of traditional cooking oil and looking for a delicious way to lose weight, then keep exploring this eBook!

Coconut Oil Recipes

Unlike normal cooking oil (hazelnut/canola oil), coconut oil contains saturated fat content but it is not harmful for health. On the other hand, scientists have confirmed the fact that 1 tablespoon of coconut oil can give off more energy than 1 tablespoon of canola oil. Here are some easy to prepare and cook meal options for a delicious breakfast, lunch and smoothie recipes which you can make using coconut oil.

Coconut Oil Breakfast Recipes

Coco-Oil Scrambled Eggs

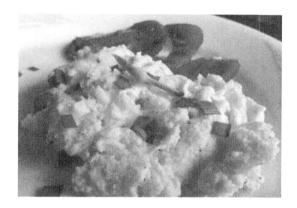

Ingredients

Coconut Oil, 1 tablespoon (for frying)

Unsweetened milk, 6 teaspoons

6 eggs

Salt, 3 pinches

Black pepper (optional), according to taste

Shredded cheese (optional)

Directions

- Start with moderately heating a large non-stick pan (make sure that the flame is set to medium).
- Whisks the eggs in a large bowl thoroughly.
- Add milk to the whisked eggs and blend together.
- Add salt and black pepper to this mixture.
- Melt the coconut oil in the preheated pan.

- Pour the whisked egg mixture in the pan and cook evenly for approximately 1 minute.
- You can sprinkle in some shredded cheese to add a cheesy flavor to scrambled eggs.

Preparation time

Less than 10 minutes

Serving Size

3 persons

Nutrition Value

Calories: 608, Fat: 44.69g, Protein: 40.59g, Carbs: 8.05g

Coconut Oil Roasted Toast

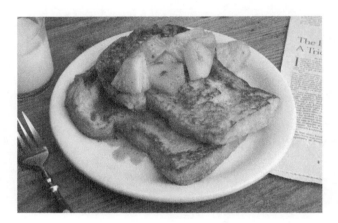

Ingredients

2 pieces of toast (brown toast or regular toast)

Coconut oil, 2 tablespoons

Directions

- The first important thing is the choice of toast. Make sure that it is not bread.
- Coat both sides of the toast with coconut oil.
- Put the oil coated toast in toaster.
- Serve warm with tea or coffee.

Preparation Time

5 minutes

Serving Size

1 person

Nutrition Value

Calories: 64, Fat: 0.88g, Protein: 1.98g, Carbs: 11.97g

Roasted Potatoes with Coco-Oil

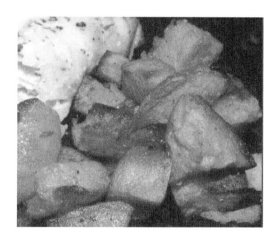

Ingredients

Sweet potatoes, 1.75 pounds

Brown sugar (optional), 2 teaspoons

Organic coconut oil (virgin), 1.5 tablespoons

Common salt, 1.5 teaspoons

Ground black pepper, a pinch

Directions:

- Peel and dice sweet potatoes.
- Preheat the oven to 370°F.
- Melt the organic coconut oil over medium flame in a non-sticking frying pan.
- Toss diced potatoes, salt, pepper and sugar in a large bowl.
- Pour the melted coconut oil over potatoes and mix all the ingredients together.
- Spread the greased potatoes in a baking dish and put it in the preheated oven for about 1 hour.
- Take out the baked potatoes and season with your favorite sauce.

Preparation Time

1 hour 10 minutes

Serving Size

2-4 persons

Nutrition Value

Calories: 361.3, Fat: 3g, Protein: 6.2g, Carbs: 88.7g

Coconut Oil Waffles

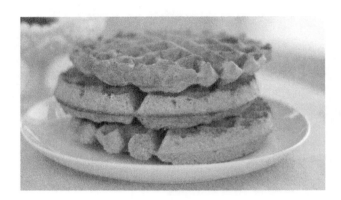

Ingredients

2 large brown eggs

Organic cereal flour, 2 cups

Common salt, a pinch

Baking powder, 4 teaspoons

Organic coconut oil, 0.5 cup

Sugar, 1 tablespoon

Directions

- Whisk the eggs thoroughly.
- Add all the ingredients to whisked eggs and keep beating to blend well.
- Heat the waffle iron over a medium flame.
- Pour more than half of the batter onto the iron.
- Close the lid of the iron and leave for 5 minutes.
- Take out the waffles as soon as the steaming stops.

- Serve with honey or maple syrup.

Preparation Time

10 minutes

Serving size

1 person

Nutrition Value

Calories: 453, Fat: 28g, Protein: 9g, Carbs: 43g

Coconut Oil Bison Burgers

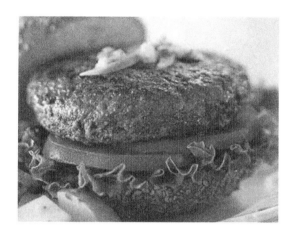

Ingredients

4 cereal buns (preferably unsweetened)

Common salt, 1 teaspoon

Organic coconut oil, 1 tablespoon

1 large egg

Pepper, according to taste

Minced garlic, 2 teaspoons

Grass-fed bison, 1.5 lbs

Directions

- De-frost the bison (if frozen).

- Whisk egg in a large bowl and add coconut oil, bison, salt, pepper and minced garlic in the bowl.
- Divide the mixture into 4 sections and fry with coconut oil.
- Heat each side for about 3 minutes.
- Sandwich the fried egg into buns and serve with your favorite topping.
- You can season it with tomato or garlic sauce.

Preparation Time

10 minutes

Serving Size

4 persons

Nutrition Value

Calories: 190, Fat: 11g, Protein: 23g, Carbs: 0g

Coconut Oil Banana Bread

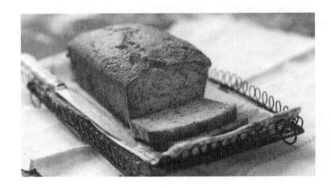

Ingredients

2 large sized bananas

Normal flour, 1.5 cups

Organic coconut oil, 0.5 cup

Cream cheese/yogurt, 1 cup

Salt, 1 teaspoon

Brown Sugar, 2 teaspoons

Baking soda, 1 teaspoon

Directions

- Mix the cereal flour, common salt and baking soda in a large bowl.
- In another bowl beat coconut oil for 3 minutes and then add cream cheese to it. Keep beating for another 5 minutes.
- Add brown sugar to this mixture and blend thoroughly.
- Mash bananas, and add to this mixture.
- Blend softly until mixed well.
- Add the sugar and baking powder to this wet mixture and blend well.
- Preheat the oven over medium flame to 360°F.
- Pour this mixture in a large loaf pan and spread well.
- Put the pan in the preheated oven.
- Bake for 1 hour.
- Serve with maple syrup or honey.

Preparation Time

1 hour

Serving Size

4-6 persons

Nutrition Value

Calories: 667, Fat: 23.7g, Protein: 5.5g, Carbs: 103.4g

Coconut Oil Lunch Recipes

Coconut Oil Sautéed Shrimp

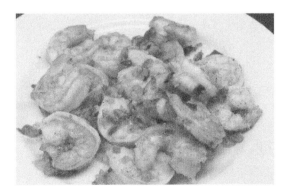

Ingredients

Coconut oil, 2.5 tbsp

1 lemon wedge

6 large green onions

Ground black pepper, 1 tsp

Minced ginger, 1 tbsp

Lemon juice, 1 tsp

2 large garlic cloves, finely minced

Kosher salt, 1 tsp

Fresh ground coriander, 1 tsp

Large shelled shrimp, 1 pound

Directions

- Melt the coconut oil in a large pan.
- Thinly slice the white part of green onions and fry for a few seconds.
- Add ginger and garlic and stir for few minutes, until the onion turns golden.
- Add coriander to the onion mixture and stir for 30 seconds.
- Add shrimp and salt to this mixture and toss these ingredients for 5 minutes.
- Keep cooking and stirring all the ingredients together until wilted.
- Dish out the fired shrimp and season with pepper and lemon juice.
- Enjoy with your favorite sauce.

Preparation Time

15 minutes

Serving Size

2-3 persons

Nutrition Value

Calories: 332.5, Fat: 19.5g, Protein: 32.1g, Carbs: 7.6g

Coconut Oil Turkey Sausage

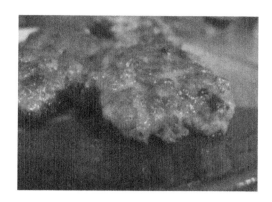

Ingredients

For Sausage:

1 large apple, finely grated

2 brown large eggs

Ground Turkey, 1 lb (preferably organic)

Crushed coconut (dried), 1 cup

For Seasoning:

Thyme, 1 tsp

Organic coconut oil, 2 tsp

Cloves, a pinch

Common salt, 1 tsp

Nutmeg, a pinch

Allspice, to taste

Onion flakes, 1 tsp

Ground black pepper, 1 tsp

Fennel seed, 1.5 tsp

Sage, 2 tsp

Garlic powder, a pinch

Directions

- Start with mixing eggs, grated apple and crushed coconut together.
- Coat the turkey with this mixture.
- Set aside the coated turkey to soak in the rub for some time.
- Meanwhile, mix all the ingredients for the seasoning together.
- Marinate the turkey with the seasoning mixture.
- Put the turkey into freezer for several hours.
- Take out the turkey and shape it into patties.
- In a large frying pan, melt the coconut oil and heat it over medium flame for a few minutes.
- Shallow fry the turkey patties in coconut oil.
- Fry each side for a few minutes until the meat is tender and juicy.

Preparation Time

5-6 hours

Serving Size

4-6 persons

Nutrition Value

Calories: 44, Fat: 2.29g, Protein: 5.33g, Carbs: 0.13g

Coconut Oil Stir Fried Chicken

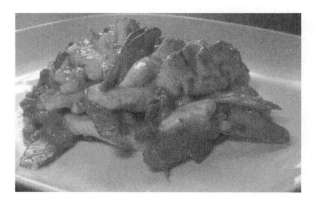

Ingredients

Organic coconut oil, ½ cup

Steamed plain rice, 2 cups

4-5 large chicken breasts

Salt, to taste

Ground pepper, to taste

2 large apples

Raw honey, ½ cup

Minced ginger, 1 tbsp

3 mushrooms (any kind), sliced

2 green onions, finely chopped

Directions

- Peel the apple and slice it into large chunks.
- Cut chicken breasts into large pieces.
- In a large frying pan, heat oil, ginger and honey over medium flame for a few minutes.
- Add chicken and apple chunks to the mixture and sauté for few minutes.
- Add sliced mushrooms to the mixture and continue tossing all the ingredients together.
- Sprinkle salt and pepper and sauté for 5-6 minutes.
- Enjoy with plain rice and chopped onions.

Preparation Time

20 minutes

Serving Size

4 persons

Nutrition Value

Calories: 340, Fat: 16g, Protein: 25g, Carbs: 25g

Coconut Oil Chicken Nuggets

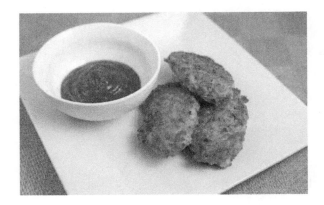

Ingredients

Coconut oil, based on pan being used to shallow fry

Organic chicken (ground), 2 pounds

Breadcrumbs or crushed cereal, 1 cup

2 large eggs

Common salt, 2 tsp

Fresh pepper, to taste

Red pepper (crushed flakes), 1 tsp

Chili powder, 2.5 tsp

Crushed garlic powder, 1 tsp

Fresh onion powder, 1 tsp

Directions

- Mix all the dry ingredients in a large bowl. Add eggs and breadcrumbs to the mixture and blend well.
- Make sure the mixture is not sticky (add more crumbs if it is).
- Slice chicken into strips, coat with mixture.
- Melt the coconut oil in a large frying pan for few minutes over a medium flame.
- Fry sliced chicken coated with all ingredients in coconut oil for few minutes.
- Dish out the chicken when it's golden brown.
- Enjoy with sauce.

Preparation Time

10 minutes

Serving Size

8 persons

Nutrition Value

Calories: 59, Fat: 4g, Protein: 3.8g, Carbs: 2.5g

Cheesy Rice with Coconut Oil

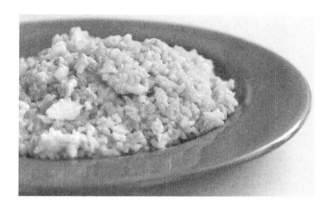

Ingredients

2 large brown eggs

Salt, to taste

Steamed brown rice, 2-3 cups

Organic coconut oil, 4 tbsp

Cheddar cheese (shredded and sharp), 4 oz

Directions

- Melt coconut oil in a frying pan over medium flame.
- Whisk brown eggs in a large bowl.
- Add steamed rice to the heated oil and stir well.
- Set the fried rice to the edges of the frying pan.
- Pour whisked eggs in the center of the pan.
- When eggs are scrambled, spread the fired rice all over.
- Sprinkle shredded cheese, salt and pepper.

- Fold the eggs in a bowl. Enjoy warm.

Preparation Time

10 minutes

Serving Size

4 persons

Nutrition Value

Calories: 333, Fat: 12.34g, Protein: 41.7g, Carbs: 12.5g

Lettuce Wraps with Coconut Oil

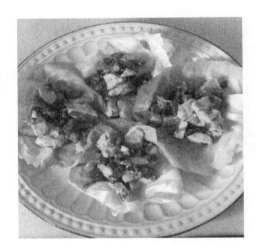

Ingredients

3 large chicken breasts (sliced into small cubes)

Organic coconut oil, 2 tbsp

Common salt, to taste

Fresh black pepper, to taste

1 fresh ginger, thinly sliced

Finely ground red pepper flakes, 1 tsp

3 fresh garlic cloves, finely chopped

1 diced green pepper

4 green onions, green and white part finely chopped

1 pack of black button mushrooms (optional)

Lettuce leaves

Gluten free tamari, 3 tbsp

Directions

- Melt the coconut oil in a frying pan for a few minutes over medium flame.
- Add garlic and ginger to the oil and fry for few seconds.
- Add chicken pieces and pepper flakes to the mixture.
- Cook the chicken for 7 minutes until tender.
- Add sliced mushrooms and green pepper to the chicken mixture and sauté for 2 minutes.
- Sprinkle tamari over the fried chicken and dish out.
- Add vegetables or beans if you like and fry them with the chicken.
- Season with any sauce.
- Serve over lettuce leaves,

Preparation Time

15 minutes

Serving Size

4 persons

Nutrition Value

Calories: 510, Fat: 10g, Protein: 28g, Carbs: 69g

Coconut Oil Dinner Recipes

Ginger Garlic Chicken

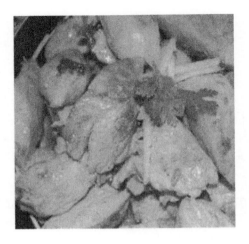

Ingredients

Chili garlic sauce, ½ cup

Organic coconut oil, 2 ½ tbsp

Fresh garlic (pressed), 3 tsp

1 large fresh ginger

3 large chicken breast pieces (boneless and sliced into halves)

Directions

- Start with cutting the chicken into thin slices.
- Peel the ginger and chop it finely.
- In a medium sauce pan, heat the coconut oil over medium flame.
- Fry sliced ginger and garlic in the coconut oil for 30 seconds.
- Add chicken slices to the melted oil and toss all the ingredients together.
- Pour chili garlic sauce over the chicken and cook for 10 to 15 minutes over low flame.
- When the meat turns golden and juicy, dish it out and enjoy.

Preparation Time

25 minutes

Serving Size

4 persons

Nutrition Value

Calories: 222, Fat: 10.5g, Protein: 20.7g, Carbs: 10.3g

Coconut Thai Steak

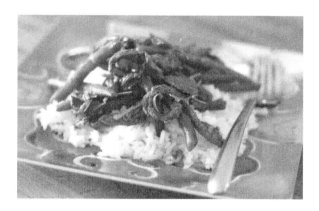

Ingredients

Coconut oil (preferably organic), 1 tbsp

Steam Rice (plain), 1 cup

Skirt Steak (very thinly sliced), ¾ pounds

Freshly chopped basil leaves, ¾ cup

Beans (preferably green and trimmed), 1 pound

Soy sauce (or fish sauce), 3 tbsp

4 large garlic cloves, minced

3 inches ginger root (peeled and very finely chopped into thin sticks)

Directions

- In a very large pan melt the coconut oil and heat over medium flame.
- Fry the steak in the coconut oil, toss gently and continue stirring until the steak turns brown, tender and juicy.
- Dish out the cooked steak and add beans, garlic and ginger to the oil.
- Fry for 6-7 minutes until the ingredients turn golden.
- Coat the fried chicken with sauces and fry for less than a minute with beans.
- Dish out quickly and enjoy with plain rice.

Preparation Time

25 minutes

Serving Size

4 persons

Nutrition Value

Calories: 190, Fat: 8g, Protein: 21g, Carbs: 10g

Coconut Fried Rice with Red Beans

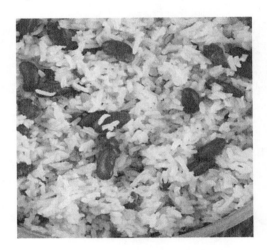

Ingredients

Coconut oil (organic), 2 teaspoons

1 complete scotch of fresh pepper (not ground or chopped)

1 large clove of fresh garlic, peeled and crushed

Unsweetened coconut milk (light), 13.5 ounces can or 1 ½ cups

1 large onion, peeled and finely chopped

Distilled water, 2 ½ cups

1 large scallion, finely chopped

Common salt, to taste

Freshly ground black pepper, to taste

Red beans (thoroughly rinsed), 15 ½ ounces can

Raw rice (plain and long grain), 2 ½ cups

Directions

- In a medium sized pan, melt coconut oil and heat over small flame for a few minutes.
- Add chopped and peeled garlic, onion and scallion to the heated oil.
- Sauté for 5 minutes until the ingredients turn light golden.
- Add red beans and rice to the oil and stir well for few minutes.
- Pour coconut milk and keep folding.
- Sprinkle salt, black pepper and scotch pepper over the rice and keep stirring.
- Heat the mixture until the coconut milk starts boiling.
- At this point cover with the lid of the pan, reduce the flame intensity and allow the mixture to simmer for 30 minutes.
- Turn off the flame and leave it covered for a few additional minutes.
- Dish out in a large plate and enjoy.

Preparation Time

35 minutes

Serving Size

10 persons

Nutrition Value

Calories: 192.4, Fat: 3g, Protein: 4.9g, Carbs: 35.4g

Coconut Oil Desert Recipes

Coconut Oil French Toast

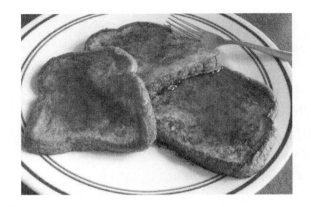

Ingredients

Plain bread (sugar or sugar free), 12 slices

Organic coconut oil, as per requirement

Vanilla essence, 1 tsp

Common salt, a pinch

Coconut milk (preferably skimmed), 1 cup

1 large banana

Fresh milk, 1 cup

Cinnamon, to taste

Cornstarch (good quality), 1.5 tsp

Nutmeg, a pinch

Directions

- Brush the pan with coconut oil and heat over small flame.
- Blend all the ingredients (except plain bread slices) in a bowl or blender.
- Pour the blended mixture in a flat dish.
- Coat both sides of every slice with the mixture.
- Heat the coated slice over lightly heated pan.
- Dish out when the slice turns golden.

- Serve with honey or maple syrup.

Preparation Time

10 minutes

Serving Size

6 persons

Nutrition Value

Calories: 377.2, Fat: 10.7g, Protein: 15.6g, Carbs: 59g

Coconut Oil Walnut Pancake

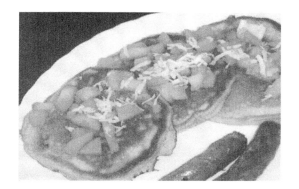

Ingredients

For Pancakes:

Finely shredded coconut (dried), ½ cup

Skimmed or non-skimmed milk, ½ cup

Organic coconut oil, as per requirement

Finely chopped walnuts, ½ cup

Baking soda, ½ tsp

Pastry flour (preferably wheat), 1 cup

Plain yogurt (good quality), 1 cup

Cinnamon, a pinch

Common salt, to taste

Baking powder, ½ tsp

4 large brown eggs

Apple topping, ½ cup

For Apple Topping:

2 large sized red apples, diced but not minced

White sugar, 2 tbsp (or add more according to taste)

Cinnamon, a pinch

Grass-fed fine quality butter, 2 tbsp

Distilled water, 1 tbsp

Vanilla essence, 1 tsp

Directions

- Start with preparing apple topping.
- Take small bowl or sauce pan and mix all the ingredients for apple sauce in the bowl.
- Add more water if needed and heat the mixture on a low flame.
- Stir the mixture well but don't boil.
- Dish out the sauce when apples are soft and blended.
- Let the sauce cool down and start preparing for pancakes.
- Mix the first five ingredients for pancakes together and set aside.
- In a bowl, whisk eggs together and add plain yogurt and skimmed milk.
- Add rest of the dry ingredients and keep blending the mixture.
- Make sure that the batter is lumpy.
- Add ½ cup of the apple sauce, crushed coconut and sliced walnuts and blend well.
- Pour the egg batter in a preheated and greased iron skillet.
- Make sure that the pancake size is not too thick.
- As soon as the top of it starts swelling, flip the batter to the other side.
- Enjoy with honey or maple syrup.

Preparation Time

20 minutes

Serving Size

4 persons

Nutrition Value

Calories: 208, Fat: 8g, Protein: 8g, Carbs: 3g

Coconut Oil Chocolate Candies

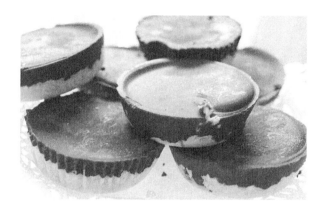

Ingredients

Organic coconut oil, half cup

Dark chocolate powder, half cup

Vanilla or strawberry extract, 1 tsp

Raw honey, 2 tbsp

Optional Ingredients

Maca powder 1 tbsp

Orange juice, 2 tsp

Dry fruits, as per choice

Dried coconut powder, 2 tbsp

Directions

- In a small sauce pan, melt the coconut oil over low flame.
- Add honey to the melted oil and mix well.

- Add dark chocolate powder and all the additional ingredients to the mixture and fold.
- Pour the mixture into an ice cube tray.
- Put the tray in the refrigerator or for 30 minutes in freezer.
- The setting time depends on the temperature of the coconut oil.
- Take out the settled candies and serve with dried coconut.

Preparation Time

10 minutes

Serving Size

20 persons

Nutrition Value

Calories: 56.4, Fat: 5.6g, Protein: 0.2g, Carbs: 2.3g

Coconut Oil Almond Cake

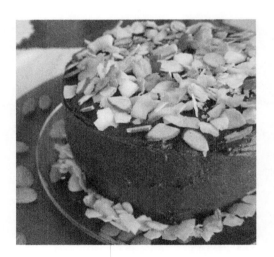

Ingredients

Organic coconut oil (good quality), 1 cup

White sugar, 2.5 tbsp

1 cup almond, finely chopped (unpeeled)

Milk (preferably unsweetened), 1 cup

4 large brown eggs

Common salt, ½ tsp

Fresh nutmeg (grated), ½ tsp

Lime zest

All-purpose cooking flour, 1 ½ cups

Fine quality baking powder, 1 ½ tsp

Directions

- Start with preheating the oven to 360°F.
- Grease a rectangular shaped cake pan with coconut oil.
- In a large bowl, mix 2 tablespoons of sugar and water together and stir until dissolved.
- Add finely chopped almonds to the sugar water and set aside for topping.
- In a large pan, melt the coconut oil over medium flame and pour into a large bowl.
- Add sugar, lime zest, eggs and milk to the melted oil and blend well.
- Mix the remaining dry ingredients in another bowl until blended uniformly.
- Combine the dry and wet mixture of ingredients together and fold thoroughly.
- Pour the batter into the greased cake pan and smooth it with a flat spatula.
- Sprinkle the sugar coated almond topping in the batter and put it in the oven.
- Bake for 60 minutes until the cake turns golden.
- Check by inserting a toothpick. If it comes out clean then your cake is ready to be served.
- Take out from the oven, leave for 10 minutes and dish out.

Preparation Time

1 hr 20 minutes

Serving Size

10 persons

Nutrition Value

Calories: 302, Fat: 66g, Protein: 7.7g, Carbs: 52.3g

Coconut Oil Granola Bars

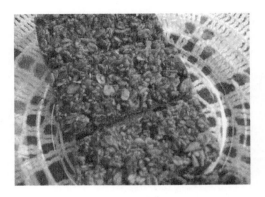

Ingredients

Sesame seeds (fresh), ¾ cup

Organic coconut oil, 1 cup

Raw honey or maple syrup, ¾ cup

Fresh peanut butter, 1 cup

Oats, 2 ½ cups

Dried coconut (unsweetened), 1 cup

Fine quality raisins, 1 cup

Flax seeds, ½ cup

Directions:

- In a medium sized frying pan, melt coconut oil over low flame.
- Add honey and peanut butter to the oil and stir well.
- Pour this mixture in a bowl and add crushed coconut, sesame seed, raisins and flax seeds.
- Fold until blended uniformly.
- Spread the mixture into a flat tray.
- Refrigerate for two hours.
- Cut the mixture into bars and enjoy.

Preparation Time

2 hrs 10 minutes

Serving Size

15 persons

Nutrition Value

Calories: 356.8, Fat: 21.3g, Protein: 9.1g, Carbs: 37.3g

Coconut Oil Snacks Recipes

Curried Popcorn with Coconut Oil

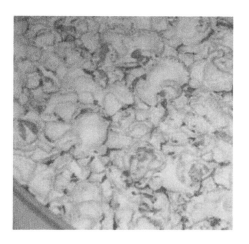

Ingredients

Organic coconut oil, 4 tablespoons

Popped popcorn (unflavored), 1 gallon

2 large garlic cloves, peeled and minced

Chili sauce, to taste

Fresh cumin, ½ teaspoon

Flavored curry powder, 1 teaspoon

Fresh turmeric (ground), 1 teaspoon

Directions

- In a small frying pan, melt the coconut oil over medium/small flame.
- Sprinkle curry powder, salt, turmeric and minced garlic and stir well.
- Keep stirring for 1 minute.
- Reduce the flame and let the mixture simmer for less than 1 minute.

- Add chili sauce to the mixture and immediately pour over unflavored popped popcorn.
- Stir for a few seconds and dish out.

Preparation Time

10 minutes

Serving Size

1 gallon

Nutrition Value

Calories: 627, Fat: 45.9g, Protein: 8.2g, Carbs: 51.8

Roasted Cashews

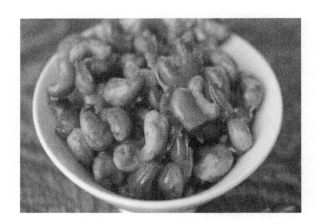

Ingredients

Fine quality organic coconut oil, 2 ½ tsp

Raw honey, ½ cup

Common salt, to taste

Smoked and fresh paprika powder, ½ tsp

Freshly ground cayenne pepper, ½ tsp

Dried coconut sugar, 2 ½ tbsp

Raw and unsalted cashews, 2 cups

Directions

- Preheat oven to 370°F.
- In a small bowl, mix coconut oil and honey together.
- Add paprika, common salt and ground pepper to the mixture.
- Add raw cashews in the coconut oil and honey mixture and fold well to coat cashews with the mixtures.
- Set this mixture aside and in another small bowl mix coconut sugar, a pinch of common salt and pepper.
- Sprinkle this powdered mixture on the honey coated cashews and toss well.
- Spread cashews in a baking dish and put it in the preheated oven for 15 minutes.
- Toss cashews after every few minutes to cook well from all sides.
- Remove the baking tray from the oven and let the cashews cool at room temperature.

Preparation Time

25 minutes

Serving Size

6 persons

Nutrition Value

Calories: 480, Fat: 35g, Protein: 14g, Carbs: 34g

Coconut Milk Recipes

Coconut Milk Breakfast Recipes

Coconut Macaroons Pancakes

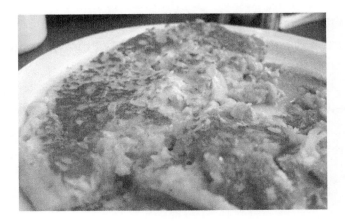

Ingredients

Good quality coconut milk (organic), 1 whole can

White sugar, ½ cup for syrup and 2 tbsp for pancakes

Unsweetened dried coconut (finely crushed), 3 ½ cups

All purpose baking powder, 2 tsp

All purpose white flour, ½ cup

Common salt, a pinch

3 large brown eggs

Butter, 2 tsp (for one pancake)

Directions

- Start with heating the coconut milk for 1-2 minutes.
- In a bowl, blend ½ tbsp sugar in warm coconut milk and stir well until dissolved completely.
- In another large bowl, mix flour, salt, and 1/2 cup sugar and baking soda together.
- Pour the sweetened coconut milk in the bowl of dry mixture and fold well.
- In a separate bowl, whisk eggs until fluffy and add the rest of the ingredients to it.

- Mix all the ingredients thoroughly and set aside.
- Heat a small frying over medium flame and melt butter.
- Pour the mixture of one pancake in the pan.
- Change sides after a few minutes and check the tenderness by lifting with a flat spatula.
- Serve with honey or maple syrup.

Preparation Time

20 minutes

Serving Size

4 persons

Nutrition Value

Calories: 79.8, Fat: 4.6g, Protein: 1.6g, Carbs: 8.7g

Coconut Milk Mango Porridge

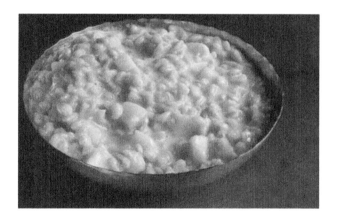

Ingredients

Unsweetened coconut milk, 13 oz. (approx 2 cans)

2 mangoes (peeled and diced), medium sized

Porridge (any cereal), 2 cups

Crushed coconut or coconut extract, ½ tsp

Brown sugar (crushed), 1/3 cup

Common salt, according to taste

Directions

- Mix the porridge with unsweetened coconut milk in a medium bowl and mix well.
- Heat this mixture over medium flame in a small pan.
- Add salt and sugar and stir.
- Keep heating for 10 minutes and stir occasionally.
- Turn the flame low and let the porridge blend well with the coconut milk.
- Dish out the porridge when all the coconut milk is absorbed.
- Enjoy with sliced mangoes.

Preparation Time

1 hour 20 minutes

Serving Size

4-6 persons

Nutrition Value

Calories: 640, Fat: 38g, Protein: 10g, Carbs: 77g

Coconut Milk Oatmeal

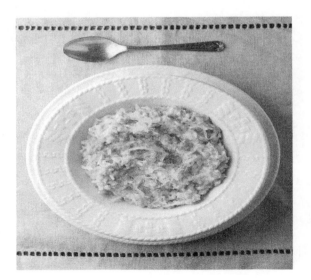

Ingredients

Organic coconut milk (preferably unsweetened), 2 ½ cups

Chopped almond (add any dry fruit of your choice), ½ cup

Cereal oatmeal, 1 cup

Flaked coconut (sweetened or unsweetened), ½ cup

Dried coconut powder, for garnishing

Raw honey, 2 tbsp for dressing

Lime juice, 1 tbsp

Directions

- In a medium sized pan, heat coconut milk and bring it to simmer.
- At this point, add oatmeal and stir for 10-15 minutes.
- When the oatmeal is tender, add flaked coconut and chopped almonds.
- Turn off the flame when all the ingredients are well combined.
- Add the lime juice to oatmeal before dishing out.
- Dress with honey and crushed coconut.

Preparation Time

20 minutes

Serving Size

2 persons

Nutrition Value

Calories: 379, Fat: 10.4g, Protein: 11.4g, Carbs: 63.1g

Gluten Free Coconut Milk Bars

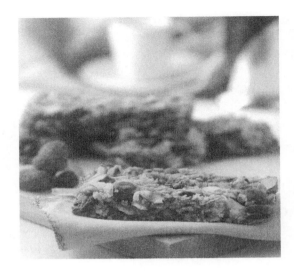

Ingredients

Fat free coconut milk, 13 ounces (or 1 full can)

Rolled oats (preferably gluten free), 2 1/3 cups

Corn starch, 2 ½ tbsp (use tapioca starch if corn is not available)

Thinly chopped almonds, 1 cup

Maple syrup or raw agave, ¾ cup

Pumpkin or sunflower seeds (roasted), 1 cup

Mixed and frozen dry fruits, 2 oz

Common salt, a pinch

Sweetened and dried coconut flakes, 1 cup

Dark chocolates (syrup or chunks), 1 cup

Directions

- Preheat the oven to 280 °F.
- Brush the baking tray with butter or cooking oil.
- Take a large bowl and mix rolled oats, sliced almonds, coconut flakes, frozen fruits, seeds and dark chocolate together and set aside.
- Take a small bowl and mix the maple syrup, coconut milk and starch together.
- Pour the wet mixture into the dry mixture bowl and blend well.

- Set aside for a few minutes and then spread the mixture into the greased baking tray.
- Put the tray in the preheated oven and bake for 50 minutes.
- Check the doneness by inserting a knife in the center of the pan.
- If the knife comes out clean, then take out the baking tray and divide the baked product into 12 bars.
- Let it cool and enjoy.

Note: you can store these bars at room temperature for up to 1 week.

Preparation Time

1 hour 25 minutes

Serving Size

12 bars

Nutrition Value

Calories: 219.9, Fat: 19g, Protein: 5.2g, Carbs: 9.7g

Coconut Milk Lunch Recipes

Chicken Curry with Coconut Milk

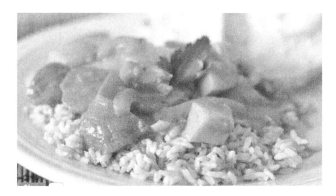

Ingredients

Skimmed coconut milk (light), 14 ounces or 1 large can

Boneless chicken breasts (sliced into thin strips), 2 lbs

Plain brown or jasmine rice (steamed), 1 ½ cups

Brown sugar (crushed), 3 tbsp

Common salt, 1 pinch

Certified tomato sauce, 8 ounces or 1 can

Freshly ground pepper, ½ tsp

Fresh Italian style tomatoes stew (organic), 14 ounces

Vegetable or sunflower oil, 2 tbsp

4 large potatoes, roughly sliced into big chunks

Paprika powder (or cayenne powder for stronger taste), 1 ½ tbsp

2 large cloves of garlic, crushed

1 small onion, finely chopped

Directions

- Season the sliced chunks of chicken breasts with pepper and salt and set aside for a few minutes.
- In a large sauce pan, heat vegetable oil, paprika powder and curry powder together until mixed well.
- As soon as the simmering begins, add sliced onions and minced garlic to the pan.
- Keep stirring for 10 minutes until the onions turn golden.
- Add the marinated chicken to this mixture and turn the flame low.
- Toss all the ingredients together for 15 minutes until the chicken is golden, tender and juicy.
- In the same pan add sliced potatoes, tomato stew, sauce and sugar and mix well to combine
- Cover with the lid of the pan and turn the flame very low.
- Leave the sauce to simmer.
- As the curry starts to thicken, dish out the chicken.
- Serve with steamed jasmine rice.

Note: you can also choose to add chili garlic sauce if you like it spicy.

Preparation Time

1 hr 20 minutes

Serving Size

4 persons

Nutrition Value

Calories: 800, Fat: 37g, Protein: 57g, Carbs: 67g

Coconut Crab Cakes

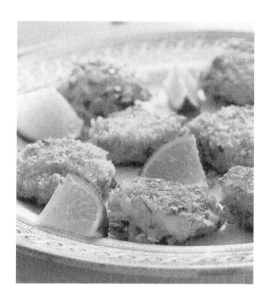

Ingredients

Fresh coconut milk, ½ cup

Red jalapeno, seeded and diced, 1 tbsp

Vegetable or canola oil, 5 tbsp

Green jalapeno, seeded and diced, 1 tbsp

Dried crumbs of brown bread, 1 cup for coating

2 ripe scallions, both white and green parts finely sliced, ½ cup

Crabmeat (lumped and picked over), 9 ounces (1 ½ cups approx)

Freshly ground ginger powder or minced ginger, 1 tbsp

Common salt, according to taste

Cilantro, roughly sliced, 2 ½ tbsp

1 large brown egg, whisked

2 large lemons, sliced into four, for serving

Directions

- In a large bowl, toss chopped scallions, ginger powder, salt and red and green jalapeno together.
- Add whisked egg and coconut milk to the mixture and whisk together until well-combined.
- Coat the crabmeat with this mixture and leave for few minutes.
- Fold the marinated crabmeat in breadcrumbs and spread in a greased baking tray.
- Cover the tray with a thin plastic sheet.
- Put the tray in the refrigerator for 30 minutes.
- Meanwhile, in a non-stick frying pan, heat vegetable oil over small flame.
- Re-coat meat slices with breadcrumbs and fry in batches.
- Flip the side after 2 minutes when the meat starts turning golden brown.
- Dish out when all sides are done.
- Enjoy with sliced lemons.

Note: Refrigerate the unused marinated crabmeat and use later.

Preparation Time

1 hr 20 minutes

Serving Size

6 persons

Nutrition Value

Calories: 240, Fat: 18g, Protein: 12g, Carbs: 10g

Coconut Thai Prawn Curry

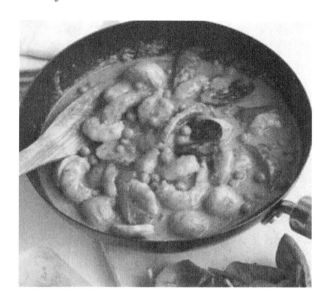

Ingredients

Skimmed and unsweetened coconut milk, 2 cans (400g each)

Fresh coriander leaves, 1 bunch

Green curry (Thai), 4 ½ tbsp

Fish sauce (Thai), 2 ½ tbsp

Lemon grass, 1 bunch fresh and finely chopped

Baby spinach, 1 small bag (100g approx)

2 large red peppers, finely chopped

Large sized prawns, 600g

New unsweetened potatoes, sliced into halves, 450g

Fresh raw peas, 220g

Chicken stock, approx 300ml

2-3 Spring onions, green and white finely chopped

1 bunch of lime leaves, roughly chopped

Fresh lime juice, 2 tbsp for serving

Directions

- In a large pan, heat oil over medium flame.
- Shallow fry the curry paste and chopped lemongrass for less than 1 minute.
- Toss slice potatoes and red pepper together and coat them with the curry paste.
- Keep cooking for 3-4 minutes.
- When the potatoes start turning golden, pour coconut milk in the pan and bring the mixture to a boil.
- Sprinkle lime leaves over it.
- Keep heating for 10-15 minutes until the mixture starts simmering.
- Add spinach and remaining ingredients (except prawns) to the coconut milk mixture, fold to combine ingredients.
- Finally add prawns and keep heating until prawns turn golden brown.
- Dress the prawn curry with lime wedges.

Preparation Time

45 minutes

Serving Size

6 persons

Nutrition Value

Calories: 324, Fat: 20g, Protein: 18g, Carbs: 20g

Coconut Milk Dinner Recipes

Coconut Milk Brazilian Chicken

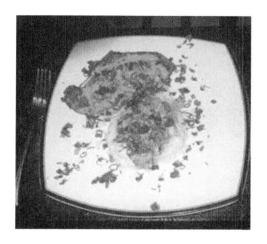

Ingredients

Skimmed coconut milk (unsweetened), 1 large can (14.5 ounces approx)

Freshly ground cumin, 1 tsp

Finely chopped fresh parsley, 1 bunch

Ground cayenne pepper or paprika powder, 1 tsp

3 large tomatoes, peeled and roughly chopped

Crushed turmeric powder, 1 tsp

2 large cloves of fresh garlic, chopped and minced

Freshly ground coriander, 1 tsp

Salt, according to taste

Black pepper, according to taste

2 red or jalapeno pepper, chopped

Olive or vegetable oil, 2 ½ tbsp

1 large onion, finely chopped

1 large fresh ginger, 1 tbsp

Boneless breast chicken pieces, 4 large pieces (sliced into big chunks)

Directions

- In a bowl mix all the spices and turmeric for marinating.
- Coat chicken with all the spices and set aside.
- Heat oil in a large skillet over medium flame.
- Cook chicken to make it tender and juicy.
- Meanwhile in a sauce pan, heat coconut milk with tomatoes, garlic, jalapeños and pepper and cook until the mixture turns into a thick cream.
- Dish out the chicken and pour the coconut cream over it.
- Enjoy with your favorite sauce.

Preparation Time

45 minutes

Serving Size

4 persons

Nutrition Value

Calories: 345, Fat: 19.9g, Protein: 11.4g, Carbs: 29.3g

Coconut Milk Chicken Stew

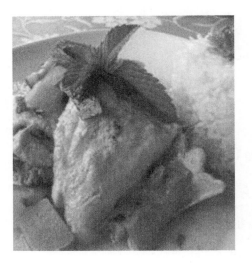

Ingredients

Unsweetened and fat free coconut milk, 1 can (14 ½ oz)

Boneless chicken breast pieces (skinless), 1 lb cut into small square chunks

Chili garlic sauce or Tabasco sauce, ½ tsp

1 large sized onion, peeled and finely chopped

Common salt, to taste

Freshly ground black pepper, to taste

Peeled and sliced potatoes, 1 ½ cups

Strong flavored curry powder, 1 tbsp

Baby carrots, sliced into small chunks, 1 cup

Cumin, 1 ½ tbsp

Green, red or lima beans, 1 packet (9 oz)

Chicken broth (fat free), 1 ½ cup

Fresh tomatoes (peeled and diced), ½ cup

Roughly torn parsley, 1 bunch for garnish

Directions

- Mix all the ingredients in a large bowl.
- Put the covered bowl in the microwave and cook for 30-40 minutes.
- Check the doneness of the chicken and dish it out.
- Enjoy with plain steamed rice.

Preparation Time

50 minutes

Serving Size

6 persons

Nutrition Value

Calories: 253, Fat: 10.4g, Protein: 21g, Carbs: 20.1g

Coconut Corn Curry

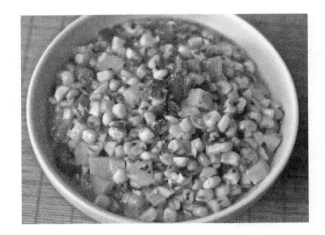

Ingredients

Coconut milk (skimmed), 3 ½ oz

Vegetable or olive oil, 4 tbsp

Cayenne pepper (freshly ground), according to taste

Seeds (preferably black mustard), 1 tbsp

Lemon juice, 2 tbsp

1 large clove of garlic, finely chopped

Common salt, according to taste

1 large potato (half cooked), diced into square chunks

Unflavored corn kernels, 2 ½ cups

Cilantro (fresh and finely chopped), diced into small pieces

Green chili (seeded and chopped), according to taste

Half bunch of mint leaves, finely chopped

1 fresh large tomato, peeled and diced

Directions

- In a large pan, heat oil over small flame.
- When the oil begins to simmer, add mustard seeds, cumin and potatoes to it.
- Keep cooking until the seeds start popping.

- At this point, add diced tomatoes, green chilies, cilantro and mint leaves and mix well.
- Keep cooking for 2-3 minutes.
- Add coconut milk and the rest of the ingredients to the mixture and blend well.
- Meanwhile in a separate pan, steam the kernels until they begin to soften.
- As the coconut milk mixture turns creamy, turn off the flame.
- Pour the mixture over steamed corn and blend well.

Preparation Time

15 minutes

Serving Size

2 persons

Nutrition Value

Calories: 150, Fat: 6g, Protein: 19g, Carbs: 20g

Coconut Milk Dessert Recipes

Coconut Milk Apple Pudding

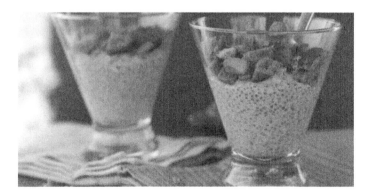

Ingredients

Coconut milk, 1 ½ cups (less than 1 can)

Seed or nut butter (preferably almond), 2 tbsp

Big chunks of unpeeled apple tartlets, 1 cup

Vanilla or strawberries extract 1 tsp

Maple syrup or raw honey (for dressing), 2 tbsp

Fresh Chia seeds, ½ cup

Direction

- In a small bowl, blend coconut milk, seed butter, maple syrup and vanilla extract with the help of an electric beater.
- Pour this fluffy mixture into a dry and airtight jar.
- Sprinkle chia seeds over it.
- Close the lid of the jar and shake vigorously.
- Refrigerate for 7-8 hours.
- Dress with roughly sliced apple tartlets.

Preparation Time

8 hours

Serving Size

3 to 4 persons

Nutrition Value

Calories: 290, Fat: 24g, Protein: 2g, Carbs: 19g

Coconut Pineapple French Toast

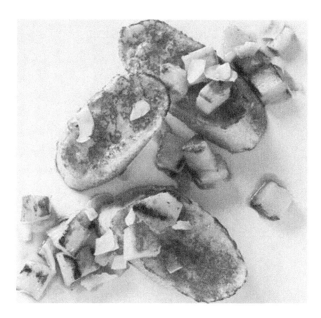

Ingredients

Unsweetened and fat free coconut milk, 1 cup

Flaked or crushed coconut, ½ cup

Brown sugar (crushed), ½ cup

Roughly chopped pineapple slices, 10-12 slices

Skimmed milk, ½ cup

4 large brown eggs

French bread, 1 loaf (divided into 15 slices)

Cooking spray, as needed

Directions

- Preheat the oven to 220°F.
- In a large bowl, combine coconut milk, skimmed milk, crushed sugar and eggs and whisk together and set aside.
- Grease a flat dish with cooking spray and heat over medium flame to make it warm.
- Dip one slice at a time in the coconut milk mixture.

- Spread the coated slices in the tray and sprinkle a few pineapple chunks over each slice.
- Put the tray in the preheated oven for 2 minutes.
- Don't change the side and dish out.
- Dress with any topping (optional).
- Enjoy.

Preparation Time

25 minutes

Serving Size

6 persons

Nutrition Value

Calories: 394, Fat: 9.1g, Protein: 11.4g, Carbs: 67.8g

Coconut Milk Coffee Cake

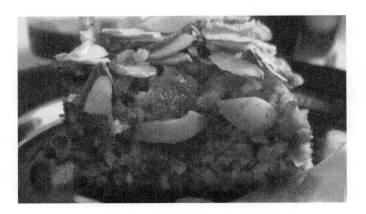

Ingredients

For cake

Good quality coconut flour, ½ cup

Unsweetened skimmed coconut milk, ½ cup

Shredded coconut (dried and unsweetened), ½ cup

Almond or nut flour, ¼ cup

Organic coconut oil (virgin and melted), ¾ cup

Common salt, to taste

Cold brew dark coffee powder, ¼ cup

Organic raw honey, ½ cup

Cinnamon powder, ¼ tsp

Coffee beans (crushed), 2 tsp

Vanilla extract, 1 tsp

Baking powder, 1 tbsp

All purpose baking soda, 1 tsp

For Dressing

Roughly chopped almonds, ½ cup

Pineapple extract or juice, 1 tbsp

Cinnamon powder, 1 tsp

Raw honey or maple syrup, 1 tsp

Organic coconut oil, 2 ½ tbsp

Common salt, according to taste

Directions

- Preheat the oven to 300°F.
- In a dry bowl, mix almonds, shredded dry coconut, baking soda, organic coconut flour and baking powder together. Mix well until all ingredients are combined.
- In another bowl mix the remaining cake ingredients and then add all the ingredients together and set aside.
- Grease a flat baking tray with oil.
- Pour the mixture of ingredients in the dish and uniformly spread.
- Put the tray in the oven and bake for half an hour.
- Check the doneness of the batter by inserting a toothpick.
- Meanwhile start preparing for the topping.
- Put a large pan over medium flame and pour coconut oil.
- Fry the crushed almonds in the oil for few minutes.
- As the almonds start turning brown, dish them out in a bowl.
- Pour maple syrup, pineapple extract and salt in the bowl and mix thoroughly.

- Take out the baked cake from the oven and coat it with the almond topping.
- Sprinkle the ground coffee powder in the end and enjoy coffee pineapple cake.

Preparation Time

50 minutes

Serving Size

6 persons

Nutrition Value

Calories: 510, Fat: 42g, Protein: 9g, Carbs: 32g

Coconut Milk Snacks Recipes

Coconut Green Smoothie

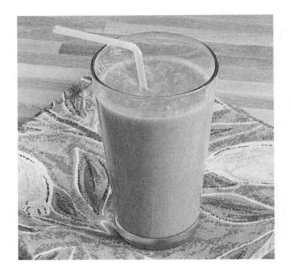

Ingredients

Coconut milk, ½ cup or ½ can

2 large bananas, unsliced and frozen

1 large peeled orange, quartered

Crushed ice, optional

Maple syrup or raw honey, according to taste

1 large lime, peeled

1-2 Kale leaf, rinsed and patted dry

Directions

- In a blender, add orange, coconut milk, kale leaf and honey and blend well.
- If the mixture is too thick for you, add water or crushed ice.
- While blending, stir with spoon occasionally to mix all the ingredients thoroughly.
- Start adding bananas to the mixture (one at a time).
- Stop the blender when the mixture is smooth.
- Chill and enjoy.

Preparation Time

15 minutes

Serving Size

4 persons

Nutrition Value

Calories: 140, Fat: 3g, Protein: 4g, Carbs: 25g

Coconut Spring Roll

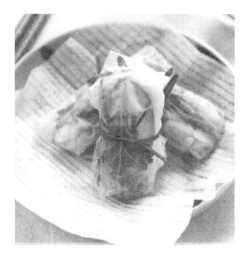

Ingredients

1 spring onion, green and white part finely chopped

Curry powder, 1 tbsp

Salt, according to taste

Fresh black pepper, according to taste

1 large capsicum, unseeded and diced

1 potato, diced and half cooked

1 cup baby carrots, finely chopped

Coconut milk, ½ cup

Vegetable oil, 2 tbsp

5 spring roll wrappers

Note: add any vegetable of your choice.

Directions

- Defrost the roll wraps.
- Shallow fry all the ingredients in vegetable oil and set aside.
- In another pan, heat coconut oil with salt, pepper and curry powder.
- When the mixture turns thick, add all the vegetables in it and blend well.
- Fill the roll wrappers with coconut milk sauté filling.
- Deep fry and enjoy.

Preparation Time

20 minutes

Serving Size

2 persons

Nutrition Value

Calories: 270, Fat: 30g, Protein: 22g, Carbs: 89g

Coconut Sauté Peanut Noodles

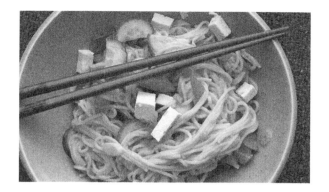

Ingredients

Plain spaghetti, 1lb or a large packet

Unsweetened and skimmed coconut milk, 1 large can (14.5 oz)

Roasted peanuts, finely crushed

Vegetable or olive oil, 2 tbsp

Soy sauce, 2 ½ tsp

Fresh chicken broth, 1 large can or 2 cups

Brown sugar (crushed), 2 tbsp

Peanut or almond butter, ½ cup

Flavored fish sauce, 2 ½ tbsp

Directions

- In a large pan of boiling water, steam the entire packet of spaghetti.
- Drain the spaghetti with cold water and set aside.
- Start preparing the sauce by heating the vegetable oil in a large skillet or wok.
- As the oil starts simmering, pour chicken broth, water and coconut milk in the skillet and stir well.
- Bring the mixture to a boil, by heating over medium flame for 10 minutes.
- Add peanut butter, soy sauce, fish sauce and sugar to the mixture and stir.
- As the mixture starts forming a creamy sauce, toss the drained noodles in it.
- Stir well and dish out after 5 minutes.
- Sprinkle crushed peanuts over the top.

Preparation Time

30 minutes

Serving Size

5 persons

Nutrition Value

Calories: 840, Fat: 53g, Protein: 38g, Carbs: 70g

Coconut Flour Recipes

Coconut Flour Breakfast Recipes

Coconut Flour Flavored Bread

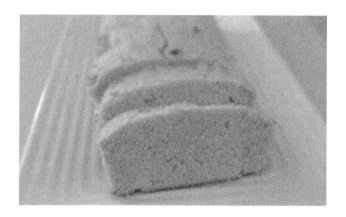

Ingredients

White coconut flour, ¾ cup

Common salt, according to taste

6 large brown eggs

Maple syrup or raw honey, 1 ½ tbsp

Unflavored butter (melted), ½ cup

Vanilla extract, 1 tsp

2 large bananas, sliced into big chunks

Directions

- Preheat the oven to 360°F.
- In a large bowl whisk eggs. Fold flour slowly into the whisked eggs.
- Add honey, melted butter, salt and vanilla extract to the egg batter.
- Add banana chunks and mix well.
- Spread the mixture in a flat baking tray and put it in the preheated oven.
- Bake for 30 minutes
- Enjoy with tea or coffee.

Preparation Time

30 minutes

Serving Size

2 persons

Nutrition Value

Calories: 93.2, Fat: 3.1g, Protein: 30g, Carbs: 2.8g

Blueberry Muffins

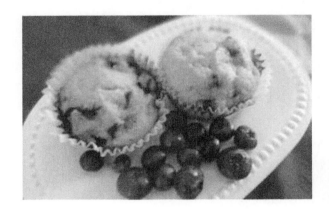

Ingredients

Coconut flour, 25 grams approx

3 medium sized eggs, only white

Blueberries, 2 ½ cups

Unflavored butter, 2 ½ tbsp

Unsweetened coconut milk, 3 tbsp

Common salt, ½ tsp

Raw honey, 1 ½ tbsp

Baking powder, ½ tsp

Vanilla extract, a few drops

Directions

- Start with preheating the oven to 300ºF.

- In a dry bowl, combine all the dry ingredients i.e. coconut flour, baking powder and salt together.
- In another large bowl, whisk egg white thoroughly and add raw honey.
- Add a few drops of vanilla extract and blend well.
- Mix all the dry and wet ingredients together.
- Add fresh and raw blueberries to the batter and gently fold the mixture.
- Pour the batter in muffin molds.
- Bake for 20 minutes.
- Cool and enjoy with your favorite topping.

Preparation Time

20 minutes

Serving Size

5 persons

Nutrition Value

Calories: 132, Fat: 9.2g, Protein: 4.4g, Carbs: 7g

Low Carb Carrot Muffins with Coconut Flour

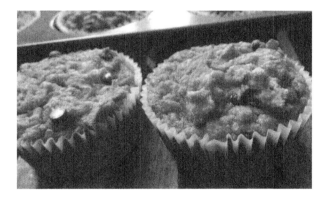

Ingredients

Coconut flour, ½ cup (25 grams approx)

5 medium sized eggs, only white

Baby carrots, 2 cups mashed

Unflavored butter, 2 ½ tbsp

Unsweetened coconut milk, 3 tbsp

Common salt, ½ tsp

Raw honey, 1 ½ tbsp

Baking powder, ½ tsp

Vanilla extract, a few drops

Cinnamon, 1 tsp

Directions

- Start with preheating the oven to 300ºF.
- In a dry bowl, combine all the dry ingredients i.e. coconut flour, baking powder and salt together.
- In another large bowl, whisk egg white thoroughly and add raw honey.
- Add a few drops of vanilla extract and blend well.
- Mix all the dry and wet ingredients together.
- Add fresh and raw carrot paste to the batter and gently fold the mixture.
- Pour the batter in muffin molds.
- Bake for 20 minutes.
- Cool and enjoy with your favorite topping.

Preparation Time

20 minutes

Serving Size

5 persons

Nutrition Value

Calories: 113, Fat: 7.2g, Protein: 3.8g, Carbs: 9.6g

Protein Waffles

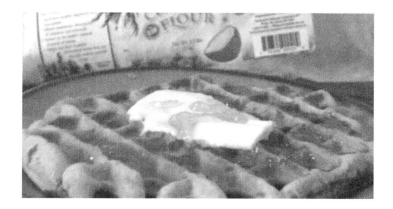

Ingredients

White coconut flour, 1 cup

8 large brown eggs

Common salt, according to taste

Unflavored melted butter (or vegetable oil), ½ cup

Vanilla extract, 1 tsp

Cinnamon powder, 1 tbsp

Directions

- In a large bowl beat all the eggs together.
- Add melted butter, cinnamon powder, common salt and vanilla extract and blend with a hand beater.
- Then add coconut flour and fold to form a thick mixture.
- Grease the waffle iron and heat it for a few minutes.
- Spread half of the batter in the iron. Cook thoroughly.
- Dish out and enjoy.

Preparation Time

10 minutes

Serving Size

1 person

Nutrition Value

Calories: 208, Fat: 4.04g, Protein: 14.5g, Carbs: 28.9g

Coconut Flour Lunch Recipes

Coconut Flour Quick Pizza

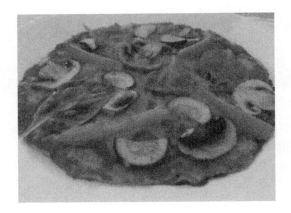

Ingredients

White coconut flour, ½ cups

4 large brown eggs

Common salt, to taste

Fresh garlic powder, to taste

Plain yogurt, 1.2 cup

Seasoning (preferably Italian), ½ tsp

Raw cheddar cheese (shredded), 2 ounces

Pizza cheese (shredded), 1 ½ ounces

Directions

- Preheat oven to 410 °F.
- In a bowl, whisk eggs until fluffy.
- Add yogurt and blend thoroughly.
- Add coconut flour and seasoning to the egg mixture and blend well to remove all the lumps.
- Set aside the coconut flour mixture for a few minutes.

- Meanwhile, brush a thin parchment paper with oil and spread the mixture over it.
- Sprinkle shredded cheese and garlic powder over it.
- Put the tray in preheated oven.
- Keep baking for 25 minutes.
- Take out and sprinkle more cheese if you want.
- Enjoy with your favorite sauce.

Preparation Time

30 minutes

Serving Size

3 persons (12 pieces)

Nutrition Value

Calories: 176, Fat: 11g, Protein: 12g, Carbs: 4.7g

Coconut Flour Tortillas

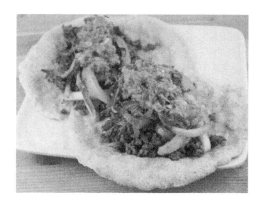

Ingredients

Filtered coconut flour, ½ cup

Common salt, according to taste

Cayenne or black pepper (ground), ½ tsp

Cumin powder, ½ tsp

Skimmed and unsweetened coconut milk, ½ cup

Egg whites, 1 cup

Garlic powder, ½ tsp

Directions

- In a large bowl, whisk egg whites together.
- Add all the ingredients to the whisked eggs and mix well.
- Set aside for a few minutes.
- In a large pan, heat some butter or oil over medium flame for a few minutes.
- Pour all the batter and turn the flame down to low.
- When the tortillas turn golden and firm, flip to the other side.
- Cook both sides over small flame for a few minutes.
- Dish out and enjoy.

Preparation Time

10 minutes

Serving Size

1 person

Nutrition Value

Calories: 46, Fat: 0.7g, Protein: 4.4g, Carbs: 1.7g

Vegetable Flat Bread

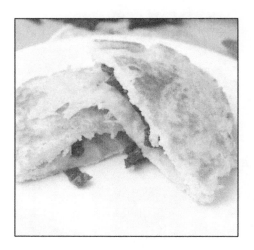

Ingredients

White coconut flour, ¾ cup

Common salt, according to taste

6 large brown eggs

Ground pepper, ½ tbsp

Unflavored butter (melted), ½ cup

Curry powder, 1 tsp

2 large carrots, sliced into big chunks

Note: add more vegetables if you want.

Directions

- Preheat the oven to 360°F.
- In a mixer whisk eggs, fold in flour.
- Add pepper, melted butter, salt and curry powder to the egg batter.
- Add carrot chunks and mix well.
- Spread the mixture in a flat baking tray and put it in the preheated oven.
- Bake for 20 minutes.
- Enjoy a low carb lunch.

Preparation Time

20 minutes

Serving Size

2 persons

Nutrition Value

Calories: 80, Fat: 3.1g, Protein: 25.8g, Carbs: 3.2g

Grain Free Coconut Vegetable Fritter

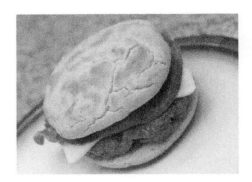

Ingredients

Filtered coconut flour, 1 tbsp

1 large brown egg

Common salt, according to taste

Fresh vegetables, of your choice

Melted butter, 1 tbsp

Directions

- Whisk eggs in a large bowl.
- Add all ingredients to the whisked eggs.
- Coat vegetables and fry in coconut oil.
- Slightly heat buns in melted butter.
- Place the vegetable fritter in the bun and enjoy.

Preparation Time

10 minutes

Serving Size

1 person

Nutrition Value

Calories: 180, Fat: 13g, Protein: 10g, Carbs: 8.5g

Low Carbs Bean Fritters

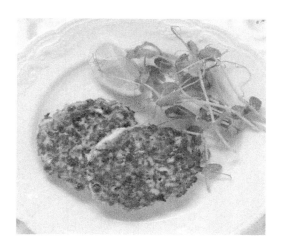

Ingredients

Peas (defrosted), 11 oz can (approx 300g)

Filtered white coconut flour, 2 tbsp

Freshly chopped parsley, ½ bunch

Common salt, according to taste

Black pepper, according to taste

2 large brown eggs

Good quality ricotta, 150g

Lime juice, 1 tbsp

Directions

- Steam peas to soften.
- In a bowl mix eggs, salt, pepper, and lime juice together.
- Add coconut flour in last and blend well.
- Mix peas in the coconut flour mixture.
- Heat a medium sized frying pan over small flame.
- Pour some of the batter in the pan.
- When the batter starts turning golden and firm, flip to the other side.
- Dish out and garnish with parsley.

Preparation Time

15 minutes

Serving Size

2 persons

Nutrition Value

Calories: 99.4, Fat: 4.6g, Protein: 8.3g, Carbs: 6g

Flour Coated Baked Chicken

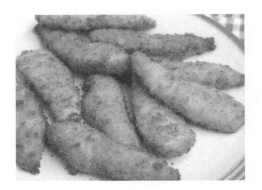

Ingredients

Filtered coconut flour, 1 ounce

Boneless chicken breast, 1 lb

Common salt, according to taste

Fresh ground black pepper, according to taste

Fresh garlic powder, 1/2 tsp

1 large organic egg

Cayenne pepper, ¼ tsp

Directions

- Preheat the oven to 270ºF.
- In a large bowl whisk egg and add all the ingredients except flour to it.
- Marinate chicken with the mixture and set aside for a few minutes.
- Coat the chicken with coconut flour and put in the oven for 40 minutes.

Preparation Time

50 minutes

Serving Size

2 persons

Nutrition Value

Calories: 171, Fat: 5.5g, Protein: 18.3g, Carbs: 11.2g

No Fry Tilapia

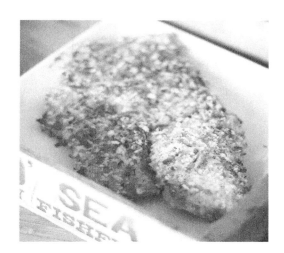

Ingredients

Filtered coconut flour, 1 ounce

Tilapia Fillets, 1 lb

Common salt, according to taste

Fresh ground black pepper, according to taste

Fresh garlic powder, 1/2 tsp

1 large organic egg

Cayenne pepper, ¼ tsp

Directions

- Preheat the oven to 300°F.
- In a large bowl whisk egg and add all the ingredients (except flour) to it.

- Marinate tilapia with the mixture and set aside for a few minutes.
- Coat the fillets with coconut flour and put in the oven for 30 minutes.

Preparation Time

40 minutes

Serving Size

2 persons

Nutrition Value

Calories: 194, Fat: 6g, Protein: 28g, Carbs: 8g

Coconut Flour Dessert Recipes

Coconut Flour Strawberry Dessert

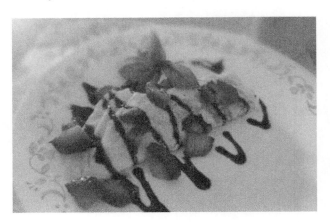

Ingredients

2 large brown eggs

White coconut flour, 2 ½ tbsp

Skimmed milk (unsweetened), ½ cup

Common salt, according to taste

Vegetable oil or melted butter, 1 tbsp

Raw honey, 1 ½ tsp

Strawberry paste or raw strawberries (diced), 1 cup

Directions

- In a large bowl, whisk eggs until beaten well.
- Add all the ingredients to the whisked eggs and blend to remove any lumps.
- In a nonstick frying pan, melt the butter over medium flame.
- Pour less than half of the batter in the pan and spread it uniformly.
- Flip the side and cook it for few seconds.
- Be careful not to break the crepe while flipping.
- Dish out and cool it down.
- Fill with strawberry paste and enjoy.

Preparation Time

15 minutes

Serving Size

2 persons

Nutrition Value

Calories: 335, Fat: 5.85g, Protein: 53g, Carbs: 20g

Coconut Flour Creamy Brownies

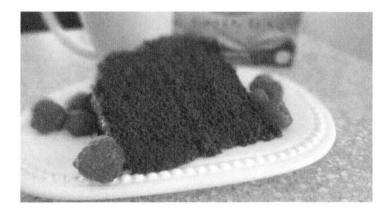

Ingredients

Coconut flour (filtered), ½ cup

10 large eggs

Dark chocolate or cocoa powder, ¼ cup

Common salt, a pinch (less than 2 tsp)

All purposed baking soda, 1 tsp

Fresh orange zest, ½ tsp

Melted butter, 1 cup

Vanilla extract, 1 ½ tbsp

Agave nectar or honey, 1 ¼ cups

Directions

- Preheat the oven to 350ºF.
- In a large bowl, mix coconut flour, baking soda and chocolate powder, and common salt together and set aside.
- In another bowl, whisk all the eggs together (preferably with hand beater).
- Add vanilla extract, honey and orange zest in to the eggs and beat well.
- Add all the dry and wet ingredients together and fold to remove any lumps.
- Grease a flat baking tray with melted butter.
- Pour the batter in it and spread uniformly.
- Put the tray in preheated oven and bake for 40 minutes.
- Allow brownies to cool down and enjoy.

Preparation Time

50 minutes

Serving Size

4 persons

Nutrition Value

Calories: 365, Fat: 2, Protein: 5g, Carbs: 53g

Coconut Flour Lamingtons

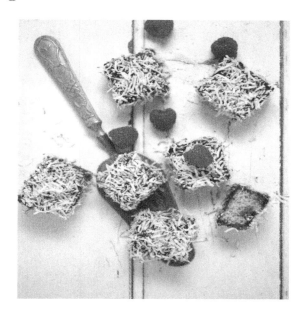

Ingredients

Coconut flour (filtered), 1 cup

6 large brown eggs

Vanilla extract, 1 tablespoon

Melted butter, ¼ cup (or coconut oil)

Salt, according to taste

Dry coconut (shredded), 1 cup for rolling

Raw honey or maple syrup, 2 ½ tbsp

Unsweetened or gluten free baking powder, 1 ½ tsp

Dried nuts, of your choice

Lamington cake mix

Apple sauce for topping

Directions

- Preheat oven to 350ºF.
- Whisk eggs in a large bowl and add maple syrup and vanilla extract.
- Set aside for a few minutes.

- Add coconut flour, baking powder, dried nuts to the mixture and keep folding.
- Add lamington cake mix to the mixture.
- Spread the mixture in a flat baking tray and put it in the oven.
- Take out after 40 minutes.
- Allow it to cool, cut into pieces, roll in dry shredded coconut, and enjoy with apple sauce.

Preparation Time

50 minutes

Serving Size

25 lamingtons

Nutrition Value

Calories: 99, Fat: 7, Protein: 2.7g, Carbs: 6g

Coconut Flour Snacks Recipes

Coconut Biscuits

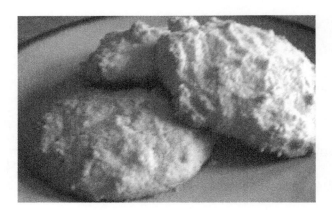

Ingredients

Coconut flour (filtered), 1 cup

Buckwheat brown flour, 2 ½ tablespoons

Lemon juice, 1 ½ tablespoon

Coconut milk (skimmed), 1 cup

1 large can of almond

Soy milk, 1 cup

Vanilla extract, 1 ½ tablespoon

Common salt, ½ teaspoon

Flax seed (finely ground), 3 tablespoons

Baking soda, 1 tsp

Stevia, few drops

All purpose baking powder, 1 tablespoon

Cooking oil or melted (unflavored) butter, 2 tablespoons

Note: 1 tsp coconut oil for greasing.

Directions

- Preheat oven to 360°F.
- Spread a thin parchment paper in a flat baking tray, grease it with coconut oil and set aside.
- Mix lemon juice with coconut milk.
- Add vanilla extract and flax seeds to the coconut milk and stir.
- Add melted butter or coconut oil to the mixture and whisk until combined well.
- Set aside the mixture for 2 minutes.
- Meanwhile start mixing the dry ingredients in another bowl.
- Mix the dry and wet mixture together and fold to remove all lumps.
- Don't mix hard, the mixture should be fluffy and soft.
- Add some skimmed milk if the mixture looks too dry.
- Set aside the biscuit dough for a few minutes.
- Fill large sized cookie moulds with the batter and align in the baking tray.
- Put the tray in the oven for 12-15 minutes until the batter turns brown.
- Remove from oven and allow it to cool.
- Enjoy.

Preparation Time

40 minutes

Serving Size

6 persons

Nutrition Value

Calories: 195, Fat: 14g, Protein: 5.8g, Carbs: 10.1g

Apple Cinnamon with Coconut Flour

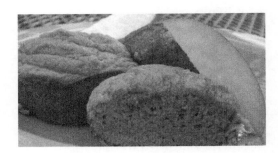

Ingredients

Coconut flour, 1 cup

2 large brown eggs

Applesauce (preferably homemade), 1 cup

Raw honey or maple syrup (optional), 1 tablespoon

Cinnamon powder, 2 ½ tbsp

Melted butter or coconut oil, ½ cup

Baking soda, 1 ½ teaspoons

Vanilla extract, 1 teaspoon

Directions

- Preheat the oven to 370°F.
- Brush the muffin tray with melted butter or coconut oil.
- Whisk all the ingredients together in a large bowl.
- Blend thoroughly until combined well and set aside for a few minutes.
- Fill small sized muffin cups with the batter and align in the tray.
- Put the tray in preheated oven and bake for 15 minutes.
- When the muffin starts to turn golden brown then take out the tray.
- Allow to cool for two minutes.
- Dress with raw honey topping and enjoy.

Preparation Time

20 minutes

Serving Size

4 persons

Nutrition Value

Calories: 360, Fat: 0.5g, Protein: 3g, Carbs: 50g

Coconut Chocolate Chip Cookies

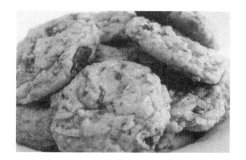

Ingredients

Coconut flour (filtered), 1 cup

Lemon juice, 1 ½ tablespoon

Coconut milk (skimmed), 1 cup

Flax seed (finely ground), 3 tablespoons

1 large bag of chocolate chips

Baking soda, 1 tsp

Buckwheat brown flour, 2 ½ tablespoons

All purpose baking powder, 1 tablespoon

Soy milk, 1 cup

Vanilla extract, 1 ½ tablespoon

Common salt, ½ teaspoon

Stevia, few drops

Cooking oil or melted (unflavored) butter, 2 tablespoons

Note: 1 tsp coconut oil for greasing.

Directions

- Preheat oven to 360ºF.
- Spread a thin parchment paper in a flat baking tray, grease it with coconut oil and set aside.
- Mix lemon juice with coconut milk.
- Add vanilla extract and flax seeds to the coconut milk and stir.
- Add melted butter or coconut oil to the mixture and whisk until combined well.
- Set aside the mixture for 2 minutes.
- Meanwhile start mixing the dry ingredients in another bowl.
- Mix the dry and wet mixture together and fold to remove all lumps.
- Don't mix too hard. The mixture should be fluffy and soft.
- Add some skimmed milk if the mixture looks too dry.
- Set aside the biscuit dough for few minutes.
- Fill large sized cookie moulds with the batter and align in the baking tray.
- Sprinkle chocolate chips over the dough.
- Put the tray in oven for 12-15 minutes until the batter turns brown.
- Remove from oven and allow it to cool.
- Enjoy.

Preparation Time

40 minutes

Serving Size

6 persons

Nutrition Value

Calories: 85, Fat: 4.7g, Protein: 5g, Carbs: 10.8g

Final Word

Coconut flour, milk and oil are not only used for cooking, but it also serves the purpose of an organic health tonic. This report includes a number of easy to cook and healthy coconut recipes which can facilitate adequate consumption of coconut on a daily basis.

Try these coconut recipes and enjoy countless health benefits!

Printed in Great Britain
by Amazon